The Essential Dash Diet Cookbook

Revamp Your Menu Without
Sacrificing Your Favourite Flavors
with Recipes for Everyone

Geneva Briggs

TABLE OF CONTENTS

INTRODUCTION

S top Hypertension, a nutritional approach to prevent hypertension (DASH). It is said to help reduce high blood pressure by following a low-protein, high-carbohydrate diet with a focus on healthy fats, fruits, vegetables and whole grains.

The DASH diet emphasizes and promotes healthy fats, fruits, vegetables, whole grains, nuts, seeds, legumes and nuts and seeds. There are several health benefits that have positive effects on blood pressure, heart disease and diabetes. Some versions of the dash diet include a low-carb - high protein and high carbohydrate - diet with an emphasis on fruits and vegetables. The strict diet allows the use of whole grains such as fruits or vegetables and whole grains.

If people with high blood pressure stick closely to the DASH diet, it can prevent the development of diabetes, heart disease, high blood pressure, high cholesterol, and other health problems. The Dash diet promotes heart health, helps with high blood pressure and prevents diabetes. Certain foods are included in the diet, but others are avoided, such as nuts, seeds, legumes and nuts and seeds.

One way to achieve this is to follow the Dietary Plan to Stop Hypertension (DASH). The Dash Diet Plan is recommended by the US Centers for Disease Control and Prevention (CDC), which says it can be used in conjunction with the "Dietary Approach to Preventing Hypertension" (DSH) diet.

The DASH diet has much more to offer than just what it does, but this is a good starting point to see how obesity is defined. There are a number of different types of obesity, such as high fat, high carbohydrate and medium fat.

Previous research has shown that following the DASH diet could help with depression, and a cookbook to lowering blood pressure with Dash issued by the NIH provides step-by-step guidance on how to switch to a DASH diet. While cutting-edge sayings are useful when it comes to improving overall mood, those who have helped lower cholesterol and blood pressure say it's more than just lowering blood pressure. In addition to a healthy diet, it also offers a number of other benefits, such as lowering cholesterol, blood pressure, heart disease, diabetes, cancer, obesity, high blood pressure and much more. The reduction in blood pressure by up to 30 percent is proven, according to the National Institutes of Health (NIH).

When the DASH diet was published in 1995, the combined effects of the diet on blood pressure, heart disease, and diabetes were revolutionary. The study results showed that the amount of sodium in the control diet was less than half of what was contained in the "DASH" diet. This study essentially ushered in a new era of research into the link between diet and chronic diseases such as diabetes and hypertension. A recent study by the National Institute of Diabetes and Digestive and Nidney Diseases (NIDD), which included a dash diet when looking at the effects of this diet on blood pressure, found that both the number of clots and blood sugar levels were significantly reduced. Their results were less original than the original study, but the results showed that there were no significant differences between the two diets in terms of cholesterol, blood sugar levels or blood pressure.

BREAKFAST

1. Creamy Apple-Avocado Smoothie

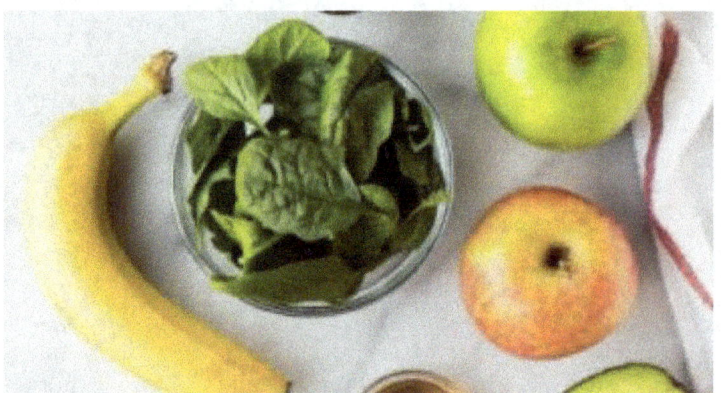

Preparation time: 15 minutes

Cooking time: 0 minutes

Servings: 2

Ingredients:

- ½ medium avocado, peeled and pitted
- 1 medium apple, chopped
- 1 cup baby spinach leaves
- 1 cup nonfat vanilla Greek yogurt
- ½ to 1 cup of water
- 1 cup ice
- Freshly squeezed lemon juice (optional)

Directions:

1. Blend all of the fixing using a blender, and blend until smooth and creamy. Put a squeeze of lemon juice on top if desired, and serve immediately.

Nutrition: Calories: 200, Fat: 7g, Sodium: 56mg, Potassium: 378mg. Carbohydrates: 27g, Fiber: 5g, Sugars: 20g, Protein: 10g

2. Strawberry, Orange, and Beet Smoothie

Preparation time: 5 minutes

Cooking time: 0 minutes

Servings: 2

Ingredients:

- 1 cup nonfat milk

- 1 cup of frozen strawberries

- 1 medium beet, cooked, peeled, and cubed

- 1 orange, peeled and quartered

- 1 frozen banana, peeled and chopped

- 1 cup nonfat vanilla Greek yogurt

- 1 cup ice

Directions:

1. In a blender, combine all of the fixings, and blend until smooth. Serve immediately.

Nutrition: Calories: 266, Fat: 0g, Cholesterol: 7mg, Sodium: 104mg, Carbohydrates: 51g, Fiber: 6g, Sugars: 34g, Protein: 15g

3. Blueberry-Vanilla Yogurt Smoothie

Preparation time: 5 minutes

Cooking time: 0 minutes

Servings: 2

Ingredients:

- 1½ cups frozen blueberries
- 1 cup nonfat vanilla Greek yogurt
- 1 frozen banana, peeled and sliced
- ½ cup nonfat or low-fat milk
- 1 cup ice

Directions:

1. In a blender, combine all of the fixing listed, and blend until smooth and creamy. Serve immediately.

Nutrition: Calories: 228, Fat: 1g, Sodium: 63mg, Potassium: 470mg, Carbohydrates: 45g, Fiber: 5g, Sugars: 34g, Protein: 12g

4. Greek Yogurt Oat Pancakes

Preparation time: 15 minutes

Cooking time: 10 minutes

Servings: 2

Ingredients:

- 6 egg whites (or ¾ cup liquid egg whites)
- 1 cup rolled oats
- 1 cup plain nonfat Greek yogurt
- 1 medium banana, peeled and sliced
- 1 teaspoon ground cinnamon
- 1 teaspoon baking powder

Directions:

1. Blend all of the listed fixing using a blender. Warm a griddle over medium heat. Spray the skillet with nonstick cooking spray.

2. Put 1/3 cup of the mixture or batter onto the griddle. Allow to cook and flip when bubbles on the top burst, about 5 minutes. Cook again within a minute until golden brown. Repeat with the remaining batter. Divide between two serving plates and enjoy.

Nutrition: Calories: 318, Fat: 4g, Sodium: 467mg, Potassium: 634mg, Carbohydrates: 47g, Fiber: 6g, Sugars: 13g, Protein: 28g

5. Scrambled Egg and Veggie Breakfast Quesadillas

Preparation time: 15 minutes

Cooking time: 15 minutes

Servings: 2

Ingredients:

- 2 eggs
- 2 egg whites
- 2 to 4 tablespoons nonfat or low-fat milk
- ¼ teaspoon freshly ground black pepper
- 1 large tomato, chopped
- 2 tablespoons chopped cilantro
- ½ cup canned black beans, rinsed and drained
- 1½ tablespoons olive oil, divided
- 4 corn tortillas
- ½ avocado, peeled, pitted, and thinly sliced

Directions:

1. Mix the eggs, egg whites, milk, and black pepper in a bowl. Using an electric mixer, beat until smooth. To the same bowl, add the tomato, cilantro, and black beans, and fold into the eggs with a spoon.

2. Warm-up half of the olive oil in a medium pan over medium heat. Add the scrambled egg mixture and

cook for a few minutes, stirring, until cooked through. Remove from the pan.

3. Divide the scrambled-egg mixture between the tortillas, layering only on one half of the tortilla. Top with avocado slices and fold the tortillas in half.

4. Heat the remaining oil over medium heat, and add one of the folded tortillas to the pan. Cook within 1 to 2 minutes on each side or until browned. Repeat with remaining tortillas. Serve immediately.

Nutrition: Calories: 445, Fat: 24g, Sodium: 228mg, Potassium: 614mg, Carbohydrates: 42g, Fiber: 11g, Sugars: 2g, Protein: 19g

LUNCH

6. Chicken and Carrot Stew

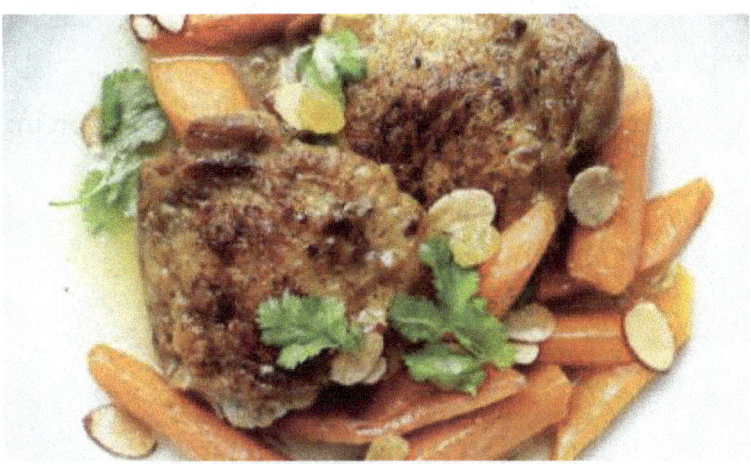

Preparation time: 15 minutes

Cooking time: 6 minutes

Servings: 4

Ingredients:

- 4 boneless chicken breast, cubed
- 3 cups of carrots, peeled and cubed
- 1 cup onion, chopped
- 1 cup tomatoes, chopped
- 1 teaspoon of dried thyme
- 2 cups of chicken broth
- 2 garlic cloves, minced
- Sunflower seeds and pepper as needed

Directions:

1. Add all of the listed ingredients to a Slow Cooker.

2. Stir and close the lid.

3. Cook for 6 hours.

4. Serve hot and enjoy!

Nutrition: Calories: 182, Fat: 3g, Carbohydrates: 10g, Protein: 39g

7. The Delish Turkey Wrap

Preparation time: 10 minutes

Cooking time: 10 minutes

Servings: 6

Ingredients:

- 1 ¼ pounds ground turkey, lean
- 4 green onions, minced
- 1 tablespoon olive oil
- 1 garlic clove, minced
- 2 teaspoons chili paste
- 8-ounce water chestnut, diced
- 3 tablespoons hoisin sauce
- 2 tablespoon coconut aminos
- 1 tablespoon rice vinegar
- 12 almond butter lettuce leaves
- 1/8 teaspoon sunflower seeds

Directions:

1. Take a pan and place it over medium heat, add turkey and garlic to the pan.
2. Heat for 6 minutes until cooked.
3. Take a bowl and transfer turkey to the bowl.
4. Add onions and water chestnuts.

5. Stir in hoisin sauce, coconut aminos, and vinegar and chili paste.

6. Toss well and transfer mix to lettuce leaves.

7. Serve and enjoy!

Nutrition: Calories: 162; Fat: 4g; Net Carbohydrates: 7g; Protein: 23g

8. Almond butternut Chicken

Preparation time: 15 minutes

Cooking time: 30 minutes

Servings: 4

Ingredients:

- ½ pound Nitrate free bacon
- 6 chicken thighs, boneless and skinless
- 2-3 cups almond butternut squash, cubed
- Extra virgin olive oil
- Fresh chopped sage
- Sunflower seeds and pepper as needed

Directions:

1. Prepare your oven by preheating it to 425 degrees F.
2. Take a large skillet and place it over medium-high heat, add bacon and fry until crispy.
3. Take a slice of bacon and place it on the side, crumble the bacon.
4. Add cubed almond butternut squash in the bacon grease and sauté, season with sunflower seeds and pepper.
5. Once the squash is tender, remove skillet and transfer to a plate.
6. Add coconut oil to the skillet and add chicken thighs, cook for 10 minutes.

7. Season with sunflower seeds and pepper.

8. Remove skillet from stove and transfer to oven.

9. Bake for 12-15 minutes, top with the crumbled bacon and sage.

10. Enjoy!

Nutrition: Calories: 323; Fat: 19g; Carbohydrates: 8g; Protein: 12g

9. Zucchini Zoodles with Chicken and Basil

Preparation time: 10 minutes

Cooking time: 10 minutes

Servings: 3

Ingredients:

- 2 chicken fillets, cubed
- 2 tablespoons ghee
- 1 pound tomatoes, diced
- ½ cup basil, chopped
- ¼ cup almond milk
- 1 garlic clove, peeled, minced
- 1 zucchini, shredded

Directions:

1. Sauté cubed chicken in ghee until no longer pink.
2. Add tomatoes and season with sunflower seeds.
3. Simmer and reduce liquid.
4. Prepare your zucchini Zoodles by shredding zucchini in a food processor.
5. Add basil, garlic, coconut almond milk to the chicken and cook for a few minutes.
6. Add half of the zucchini Zoodles to a bowl and top with creamy tomato basil chicken.
7. Enjoy!

Nutrition: Calories: 540; Fat: 27g; Carbohydrates: 13g; Protein: 59g

10. Duck with Cucumber and Carrots

Preparation time: 10 minutes

Cooking time: 40 minutes

Servings: 8

Ingredients:

- 1 duck, cut up into medium pieces
- 1 chopped cucumber, chopped
- 1 tablespoon low sodium vegetable stock
- 2 carrots, chopped
- 2 cups of water
- Black pepper as needed
- 1-inch ginger piece, grated

Directions:

1. Add duck pieces to your Instant Pot.
2. Add cucumber, stock, carrots, water, ginger, pepper and stir.
3. Lock up the lid and cook on LOW pressure for 40 minutes.
4. Release the pressure naturally.
5. Serve and enjoy!

Nutrition: Calories: 206; Fats: 7g; Carbs: 28g; Protein: 16g

DINNER

11. Lime Shrimp and Kale

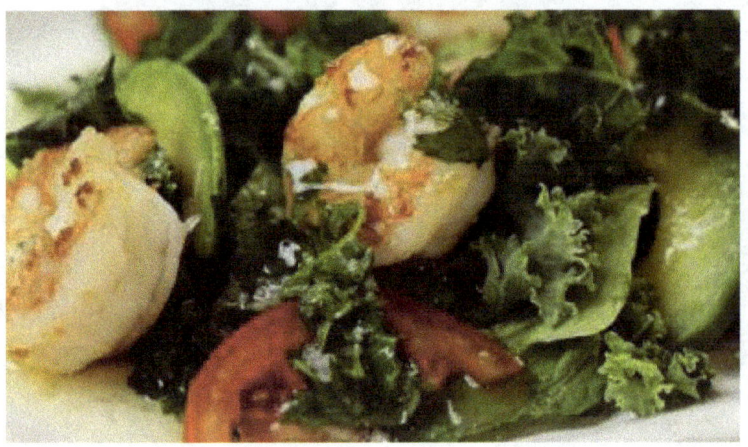

Preparation time: 10 minutes

Cooking time: 20 minutes

Servings: 4

Ingredients:

- 1-pound shrimp, peeled and deveined
- 4 scallions, chopped
- 1 teaspoon sweet paprika
- 1 tablespoon olive oil
- Juice of 1 lime
- Zest of 1 lime, grated
- A pinch of salt and black pepper
- 2 tablespoons parsley, chopped

Directions:

1. Bring the pan to medium heat, add the scallions and sauté for 5 minutes. Add the shrimp and the other ingredients, toss, cook over medium heat for 15 minutes more, divide into bowls and serve.

Nutrition: Calories: 149; Carbs: 12g; Fat: 4g; Protein: 21g; Sodium: 250 mg

12. Parsley Cod Mix

Preparation time: 10 minutes

Cooking time: 20 minutes

Servings: 4

Ingredients:

- 1 tablespoon olive oil
- 2 shallots, chopped
- 4 cod fillets, boneless and skinless
- 2 garlic cloves, minced
- 2 tablespoons lemon juice
- 1 cup chicken stock
- A pinch of salt and black pepper

Directions:

1. Bring the pan to medium heat -high heat, add the shallots and the garlic and sauté for 5 minutes. Add the cod and the other ingredients, cook everything for 15 minutes more, divide between plates and serve for lunch.

Nutrition: Calories: 216; Carbs: 7g; Fat: 5g; Protein: 34g; Sodium: 380 mg

13. Salmon and Cabbage Mix

Preparation time: 5 minutes

Cooking time: 25 minutes

Servings: 4

Ingredients:

- 4 salmon fillets, boneless
- 1 yellow onion, chopped
- 2 tablespoons olive oil
- 1 cup red cabbage, shredded
- 1 red bell pepper, chopped
- 1 tablespoon rosemary, chopped
- 1 tablespoon coriander, ground
- 1 cup tomato sauce
- A pinch of sea salt
- black pepper

Directions:

1. Bring the pan to medium heat, add the onion and sauté for 5 minutes. Put the fish and sear it within 2 minutes on each side. Add the cabbage and the remaining ingredients, toss, cook over medium heat for 20 minutes more, divide between plates and serve.

Nutrition: Calories: 130; Carbs: 8g; Fat: 6g; Protein: 12g; Sodium: 345 mg

14. Decent Beef and Onion Stew

Preparation time: 10 minutes

Cooking time: 1-2 hours

Servings: 4

Ingredients:

- 2 pounds lean beef, cubed
- 3 pounds shallots, peeled
- 5 garlic cloves, peeled, whole
- 3 tablespoons tomato paste
- 1 bay leaves
- ¼ cup olive oil
- 3 tablespoons lemon juice

Directions:

1. Take a stew pot and place it over medium heat.
2. Add olive oil and let it heat up.
3. Add meat and brown.
4. Add remaining ingredients and cover with water.
5. Bring the whole mix to a boil.
6. Reduce heat to low and cover the pot.
7. Simmer for 1-2 hours until beef is cooked thoroughly.
8. Serve hot!

Nutrition: Calories: 136; Fat: 3g; Carbohydrates: 0.9g; Protein: 24g

15. Clean Parsley and Chicken Breast

Preparation time: 10 minutes

Cooking time: 40 minutes

Servings: 2

Ingredients:

- 1/2 tablespoon dry parsley
- 1/2 tablespoon dry basil
- 2 chicken breast halves, boneless and skinless
- 1/4 teaspoon sunflower seeds
- 1/4 teaspoon red pepper flakes, crushed
- 1 tomato, sliced

Directions:

1. Pre-heat your oven to 350 degrees F.
2. Take a 9x13 inch baking dish and grease it up with cooking spray.
3. Sprinkle 1 tablespoon of parsley, 1 teaspoon of basil and spread the mixture over your baking dish.
4. Arrange the chicken breast halves over the dish and sprinkle garlic slices on top.
5. Take a small bowl and add 1 teaspoon parsley, 1 teaspoon of basil, sunflower seeds, basil, and red pepper and mix well. Pour the mixture over the chicken breast.
6. Top with tomato slices and cover, bake for 25 minutes.

7. Remove the cover and bake for 15 minutes more.

8. Serve and enjoy!

Nutrition: Calories: 150; Fat: 4g; Carbohydrates: 4g; Protein: 25g

MAINS

16. Very Wild Mushroom Pilaf

Preparation time: 10 minutes

Cooking time: 3 hours

Servings: 4

Ingredients:

- 1 cup wild rice
- 2 garlic cloves, minced
- 6 green onions, chopped
- 2 tablespoons olive oil
- ½ pound baby Bella mushrooms
- 2 cups water

Directions:

1. Add rice, garlic, onion, oil, mushrooms and water to your Slow Cooker.
2. Stir well until mixed.
3. Place lid and cook on LOW for 3 hours.
4. Stir pilaf and divide between serving platters.
5. Enjoy!

Nutrition: 156 Calories, 9.4g Protein, 12.2g Carbohydrates, 7.1g Fat, 0.8g Fiber, 7mg Cholesterol, 86mg Sodium, 365mg Potassium

17. Sporty Baby Carrots

Preparation time: 5 minutes

Cooking time: 5 minutes

Servings: 4

Ingredients:

- 1 pound baby carrots
- 1 cup water
- 1 tablespoon clarified ghee
- 1 tablespoon chopped up fresh mint leaves
- Sea flavored vinegar as needed

Directions:

1. Place a steamer rack on top of your pot and add the carrots.
2. Add water.
3. Lock the lid and cook at HIGH pressure for 2 minutes.
4. Do a quick release.
5. Pass the carrots through a strainer and drain them.
6. Wipe the insert clean.
7. Return the insert to the pot and set the pot to Sauté mode.
8. Add clarified butter and allow it to melt.
9. Add mint and sauté for 30 seconds.
10. Add carrots to the insert and sauté well.

11. Remove them and sprinkle with bit of flavored vinegar on top. Enjoy

Nutrition: 156 Calories, 9.4g Protein, 12.2g Carbohydrates, 7.1g Fat, 0.8g Fiber, 7mg Cholesterol, 86mg Sodium, 365mg Potassium

18. Garden Salad

Preparation time: 5 minutes

Cooking time: 20 minutes

Servings: 6

Ingredients:

- 1 pound raw peanuts in shell
- 1 bay leaf
- 2 medium-sized chopped up tomatoes
- ½ cup diced up green pepper
- ½ cup diced up sweet onion
- ¼ cup finely diced hot pepper
- ¼ cup diced up celery
- 2 tablespoons olive oil
- ¾ teaspoon flavored vinegar
- ¼ teaspoon freshly ground black pepper

Directions:

1. Boil your peanuts for 1 minute and rinse them.
2. The skin will be soft, so discard the skin.
3. Add 2 cups of water to the Instant Pot.
4. Add bay leaf and peanuts.
5. Lock the lid and cook on HIGH pressure for 20 minutes.
6. Drain the water.

7. Take a large bowl and add the peanuts, diced up vegetables.

8. Whisk in olive oil, lemon juice, pepper in another bowl.

9. Pour the mixture over the salad and mix. Enjoy!

Nutrition: 156 Calories, 9.4g Protein, 12.2g Carbohydrates, 7.1g Fat, 0.8g Fiber, 7mg Cholesterol, 86mg Sodium, 365mg Potassium

19. Baked Smoky Broccoli and Garlic

Preparation time: 5 minutes

Cooking time: 20 minutes

Servings: 6

Ingredients

- Cooking spray
- 1 tablespoon extra-virgin olive oil
- 3 cloves garlic, minced
- 1/2 teaspoon sea salt
- 1/4 teaspoon ground black pepper
- ½ tsp. cumin
- ½ tsp. annatto seeds
- 3 1/2 cups sliced broccoli
- 1 lime, cut into wedges
- 1 tablespoon chopped fresh cilantro

Directions:

1. Preheat your oven to 450 degrees F.
2. Line a baking sheet with foil and grease with olive oil.
3. Mix the olive oil, garlic, cumin, annatto seeds, salt, and pepper in a bowl.
4. Add in the cauliflower, carrots, and broccoli.
5. Combine until well coated.
6. Spread them out in a single layer on the baking sheet.

7. Add the lime wedges.

8. Roast in the oven until vegetables become caramelized, for about 25 minutes.

9. Take out the lime wedges and top with the cilantro.

Nutrition: 156 Calories, 9.4g Protein, 12.2g Carbohydrates, 7.1g Fat, 0.8g Fiber, 7mg Cholesterol, 86mg Sodium, 365mg Potassium

20. Roasted Cauliflower and Lima Beans

Preparation time: 5 minutes

Cooking time: 20 minutes

Servings: 6

Ingredients

- Cooking spray
- 1 tablespoon melted vegan butter/margarine
- 9 cloves garlic, minced
- 1/2 teaspoon sea salt
- 1/4 teaspoon ground black pepper
- 1 1/2 cups sliced cauliflower
- 3 1/2 cups cherry tomatoes
- 1 (15 ounce) can lima beans, drained
- 1 lemon , cut into wedges

Directions:

1. Preheat your oven to 450 degrees F.
2. Line a baking sheet with foil and grease with melted vegan butter or margarine.
3. Mix the olive oil, garlic, salt, and pepper in a bowl.
4. Add in the cauliflower, tomatoes, and lima beans
5. Combine until well coated.
6. Spread them out in a single layer on the baking sheet.
7. Add the lemon wedges.

8. Roast in the oven until vegetables become caramelized, for about 25 minutes.

9. Take out the lemon wedges.

Nutrition: 156 Calories, 9.4g Protein, 12.2g Carbohydrates, 7.1g Fat, 0.8g Fiber, 7mg Cholesterol, 86mg Sodium, 365mg Potassium

SIDES & APPETIZERS

21. Avocado, Tomato, and Olives Salad

Preparation time: 5 minutes

Cooking time: 0 minutes

Servings: 4

Ingredients:

- 2 tablespoons olive oil
- 2 avocados, cut into wedges
- 1 cup Kalamata olives, pitted and halved
- 1 cup tomatoes, cubed
- 1 tablespoon ginger, grated
- A pinch of black pepper
- 2 cups baby arugula
- 1 tablespoon balsamic vinegar

Directions:

1. In a bowl, combine the avocados with the Kalamata and the other ingredients, toss and serve as a side dish.

Nutrition: Calories 320; Protein 3g; Carbohydrates 13.9g; Fat 30.4g; Fiber 8.7g; Sodium 305mg; Potassium 655mg

22. Radish and Olives Salad

Preparation time: 5 minutes

Cooking time: 0 minutes

Servings: 4

Ingredients:

- 2 green onions, sliced
- 1-pound radishes, cubed
- 2 tablespoons balsamic vinegar
- 2 tablespoon olive oil
- 1 teaspoon chili powder
- 1 cup black olives, pitted and halved
- A pinch of black pepper

Directions:

1. Mix radishes with the onions and the other ingredients in a large salad bowl, toss, and serve as a side dish.

Nutrition: Calories 123; Protein 1.3; Carbohydrates 6.9g; Fat 10.8g; Fiber 3.3g; Sodium 345mg; Potassium 306mg

23. Spinach and Endives Salad

Preparation time: 5 minutes

Cooking time: 0 minutes

Servings: 4

Ingredients:

- 2 endives, roughly shredded
- 1 tablespoon dill, chopped
- ¼ cup lemon juice
- ¼ cup olive oil
- 2 cups baby spinach
- 2 tomatoes, cubed
- 1 cucumber, sliced
- ½ cups walnuts, chopped

Directions:

1. In a large bowl, combine the endives with the spinach and the other ingredients, toss and serve as a side dish.

Nutrition: Calories 238; Protein 5.7g; Carbohydrates 8.4g; Fat 22.3g; Fiber 3.1g; Sodium 24mg; Potassium 506mg

24. Basil Olives Mix

Preparation time: 5 minutes

Cooking time: 0 minutes

Servings: 4

Ingredients:

- 2 tablespoons olive oil
- 1 tablespoon balsamic vinegar
- A pinch of black pepper
- 4 cups corn
- 2 cups black olives, pitted and halved
- 1 red onion, chopped
- ½ cup cherry tomatoes halved
- 1 tablespoon basil, chopped
- 1 tablespoon jalapeno, chopped
- 2 cups romaine lettuce, shredded

Directions:

1. Mix the corn with the olives, lettuce, and the other ingredients in a large bowl, toss well, divide between plates and serve as a side dish.

Nutrition: Calories 290; Protein 6.2g; Carbohydrates 37.6g; Fat 16.1g; Fiber 7.4g; Sodium 613mg; Potassium 562mg

25. Arugula Salad

Preparation time: 5 minutes

Cooking time: 0 minutes

Servings: 4

Ingredients:

- ¼ cup pomegranate seeds
- 5 cups baby arugula
- 6 tablespoons green onions, chopped
- 1 tablespoon balsamic vinegar
- 2 tablespoons olive oil
- 3 tablespoons pine nuts
- ½ shallot, chopped

Directions:

1. In a salad bowl, combine the arugula with the pomegranate and the other ingredients, toss and serve.

Nutrition: Calories 120; Protein 1.8g; Carbohydrates 4.2g; Fat 11.6g; Fiber 0.9g; Sodium 9mg; Potassium 163mg

26. Cod Salad with Mustard

Preparation time: 12 minutes

Cooking time: 12 minutes

Servings: 4

Ingredients:

- 4 medium cod fillets, skinless and boneless
- 2 tablespoons mustard
- tablespoon tarragon, chopped
- tablespoon capers, drained
- 4 tablespoons olive oil+ 1 teaspoon
- Black pepper to the taste
- cups baby arugula
- small red onion, sliced
- 1 small cucumber, sliced
- tablespoons lemon juice

Directions:

1. In a bowl, mix mustard with 2 tablespoons olive oil, tarragon and capers and whisk.

2. Heat up a pan with 1 teaspoon oil over medium-high heat, add fish, season with black pepper to the taste,

and cook for 6 minutes on each side and cut into medium cubes.

3. In a salad bowl, combine the arugula with onion, cucumber, lemon juice, cod and mustard mix, toss and serve.

4. Enjoy!

Nutrition: Calories 258, Fat 12, Fiber 6, Carbs 12, Protein 18

27. Broccoli and Cod Mash

Preparation Time: 10 minutes

Cooking Time: 20 minutes

Servings: 1

Ingredients:

- 2 cups broccoli, chopped
- 4 cod fillets, boneless, chopped
- white onion, chopped
- tablespoons olive oil
- cup of water
- tablespoon low-fat cream cheese
- ½ teaspoon ground black pepper

Directions:

1. Roast the cod in the saucepan with olive oil for 1 minute per side.
2. Then add all remaining ingredients except cream cheese and boil the meal for 18 minutes.
3. After this, drain water, add cream cheese, and stir the meal well.

Nutrition: 186 calories, 21.8g protein, 5.8g carbohydrates, 9.1g fat, 1.8g fiber, 43mg cholesterol, 105mg sodium, 191mg potassium

28. Greek Style Salmon

Preparation Time: 10 minutes

Cooking Time: 10 minutes

Servings: 2

Ingredients:

- 4 medium salmon fillets, skinless and boneless
- tablespoon lemon juice
- 1 tablespoon dried oregano
- 1 teaspoon dried thyme
- ¼ teaspoon onion powder
- 1 tablespoon olive oil

Directions:

1. Heat up olive oil in the skillet.
2. Sprinkle the salmon with dried oregano, thyme, onion powder, and lemon juice.
3. Put the fish in the skillet and cook for 4 minutes per side.

Nutrition: 271 calories, 34.7g protein, 1.1g carbohydrates, 14.7g fat, 0.6g fiber, 78mg cholesterol, 80mg sodium, 711mg potassium

29. Spicy Ginger Sea bass

Preparation Time: 5 minutes

Cooking Time: 10 minutes

Servings: 2

Ingredients:

- tablespoon ginger, grated
- tablespoons sesame oil
- ¼ teaspoon chili powder
- sea bass fillets, boneless
- tablespoon margarine

Directions:

1. Heat up sesame oil and margarine in the skillet.
2. Add chili powder and ginger.
3. Then add sea bass and cook the fish for 3 minutes per side.
4. Then close the lid and simmer the fish for 3 minutes over low heat.

Nutrition: 216 calories, 24g protein, 1.1g carbohydrates, 12.3g fat, 0.2g fiber, 54mg cholesterol, 123mg sodium, 354mg potassium

30. Yogurt Shrimps

Preparation Time: 5 minutes

Cooking Time: 10 minutes

Servings: 2

Ingredients:

- pound shrimp, peeled
- 1 tablespoon margarine
- ¼ cup low-fat yogurt
- 1 teaspoon lemon zest, grated
- 1 chili pepper, chopped

Directions:

1. Melt the margarine in the skillet, add chili pepper, and roast it for 1 minute.
2. Then add shrimps and lemon zest.
3. Roast the shrimps for 2 minutes per side.
4. After this, add yogurt, stir the shrimps well and cook for 5 minutes.

Nutrition: 137 calories, 21.4g protein, 2.4g carbohydrates, 4g fat, 0.1g fiber, 192mg cholesterol, 257mg sodium, 187mg potassium

POULTRY

31. Chicken Tortillas

Preparation time: 15 minutes

Cooking time: 5 minutes

Servings: 4

Ingredients:

- 6 oz. boneless, skinless, and cooked chicken breasts
- Black pepper
- 1/3 c. fat-free yogurt
- 4 heated up whole-wheat tortillas
- 2 chopped tomatoes

Directions:

1. Heat-up a pan over medium heat, add one tortilla during those times, heat up, and hang them on the working surface. Spread yogurt on each tortilla, add chicken and tomatoes, roll, divide between plates and serve. Enjoy!

Nutrition: Calories: 190 Fat: 2 g Carbs: 12 g Protein: 6 g Sodium: 300 mg

32. Chicken with Potatoes Olives & Sprouts

Preparation time: 15 minutes

Cooking time: 35 minutes

Servings: 4

Ingredients:

- lb. chicken breasts, skinless, boneless, and cut into pieces
- ¼ cup olives, quartered
- tsp. oregano
- 1 ½ tsp. Dijon mustard
- 1 lemon juice
- 1/3 cup vinaigrette dressing
- 1 medium onion, diced
- cups potatoes cut into pieces
- cups Brussels sprouts, trimmed and quartered
- ¼ tsp. pepper
- ¼ tsp. salt

Directions:

1. Warm-up oven to 400 F. Place chicken in the center of the baking tray, then place potatoes, sprouts, and onions around the chicken.

2. In a small bowl, mix vinaigrette, oregano, mustard, lemon juice, and salt and pour over chicken and veggies. Sprinkle olives and season with pepper.

3. Bake in preheated oven for 20 minutes. Transfer chicken to a plate. Stir the vegetables and roast for 15 minutes more. Serve and enjoy.

Nutrition: Calories: 397 Fat: 13g Protein: 38.3g Carbs: 31.4g Sodium 175 mg

33. Garlic Mushroom Chicken

Preparation time: 15 minutes

Cooking time: 15 minutes

Servings: 4

Ingredients:

- 4 chicken breasts, boneless and skinless
- 3 garlic cloves, minced
- onion, chopped
- cups mushrooms, sliced
- tbsp. olive oil
- ½ cup chicken stock
- ¼ tsp. pepper
- ½ tsp. salt

Directions:

1. Season chicken with pepper and salt. Warm oil in a pan on medium heat, then put season chicken in the pan and cook for 5-6 minutes on each side. Remove and place on a plate.

2. Add onion and mushrooms to the pan and sauté until tender, about 2-3 minutes. Add garlic and sauté for a minute. Add stock and bring to boil. Stir well and cook for 1-2 minutes. Pour over chicken and serve.

Nutrition: Calories: 331 Fat: 14.5g Protein: 43.9g Carbs: 4.6g Sodium 420 mg

34. Grilled Chicken

Preparation time: 15 minutes

Cooking time: 15 minutes

Servings: 4

Ingredients:

- 4 chicken breasts, skinless and boneless
- ½ tsp. dried oregano
- 1 tsp. paprika
- 5 garlic cloves, minced
- ½ cup fresh parsley, minced
- ½ cup olive oil
- ½ cup fresh lemon juice
- Pepper
- Salt

Directions:

1. Add lemon juice, oregano, paprika, garlic, parsley, and olive oil to a large zip-lock bag. Season chicken with pepper and salt and add to bag. Seal bag and shake well to coat chicken with marinade. Let sit chicken in the marinade for 20 minutes.

2. Remove chicken from marinade and grill over medium-high heat for 5-6 minutes on each side. Serve and enjoy.

Nutrition: Calories: 512 Fat: 36.5g Protein: 43.1g Carbs: 3g Sodium 110mg

35. Delicious Lemon Chicken Salad

Preparation time: 15 minutes

Cooking time: 5 minutes

Servings: 4

Ingredients:

- lb. chicken breast, cooked and diced
- tbsp. fresh dill, chopped
- tsp. olive oil
- 1/4 cup low-fat yogurt
- tsp. lemon zest, grated
- tbsp. onion, minced
- ¼ tsp. pepper
- ¼ tsp. salt

Directions:

1. Put all you're fixing into the large mixing bowl and toss well. Season with pepper and salt. Cover and place in the refrigerator. Serve chilled and enjoy.

Nutrition: Calories: 165 Fat: 5.4g Protein: 25.2g Carbs: 2.2g Sodium 153mg

MEAT

36. Ground Pork and Kale Soup

Preparation time: 10 minutes

Cooking time: 30 minutes

Servings: 4

Ingredients:

- 1 pound pork, ground
- 3 carrots, chopped
- 4 potatoes, chopped
- 1 yellow onion, chopped
- ½ bunch kale, chopped
- 4 garlic cloves, minced
- 2 cups squash, cooked and pureed
- 2 quarts low-sodium veggie stock
- Black pepper to the taste
- 3 teaspoons Italian seasoning

Directions:

1. Heat up a pot over medium-high heat, add pork, stir, and brown for 5 minutes and transfer to a bowl.

2. Heat up the pot again over medium heat, add potatoes, onion, carrots, kale, garlic and pepper, stir and cook for 10 minutes.

3. Return beef, also add stock, squash puree and Italian seasoning, stir, simmer over medium heat for 15 minutes, ladle into bowls and serve.

4. Enjoy!

Nutrition: Calories 270, Fat 12, Fiber 6, Carbs 12, Protein 23

37. Peaches and Kale Steak Salad

Preparation time: 10 minutes

Cooking time: 12 minutes

Servings: 2

Ingredients:

- 2 peaches, chopped
- 3 handfuls kale, chopped
- 8 ounces pork steak, cut into strips
- 1 tablespoon avocado oil
- A drizzle of olive oil
- 1 tablespoon balsamic vinegar

Directions:

1. Heat up a pan with the avocado oil over medium-high heat, add steak strips, cook them for 6 minutes on each side and transfer to a salad bowl.

2. Add peaches, kale, olive oil and vinegar, toss and serve.

3. Enjoy!

Nutrition: Calories 240, Fat 5, Fiber 4, Carbs 8, Protein 15

38. Garlic Pork Meatballs

Preparation Time: 10 minutes

Cooking Time: 28 minutes

Servings: 2

Ingredients:

- 2 pork medallions
- 1 teaspoon minced garlic
- ¼ cup of coconut milk
- 1 tablespoon olive oil
- 1 teaspoon cayenne pepper

Directions:

1. Sprinkle each pork medallion with cayenne pepper.
2. Heat up olive oil in the skillet and add meat.
3. Roast the pork medallions for 3 minutes from each side.
4. After this, add coconut milk and minced garlic. Close the lid and simmer the meat for 20 minutes on low heat.

Nutrition: 284 calories, 25.9g protein, 2.6g carbohydrates, 18.8g fat, 0.9g fiber, 70mg cholesterol, 60mg sodium, 103mg potassium.

39. Fajita Pork Strips

Preparation Time: 10 minutes

Cooking Time: 35 minutes

Servings: 2

Ingredients:

- 16 oz. pork sirloin
- 1 tablespoon Fajita seasonings
- 1 tablespoon canola oil

Directions:

1. Cut the pork sirloin into the strips and sprinkle with fajita seasonings and canola oil.

2. Then transfer the meat in the baking tray in one layer.

3. Bake it for 35 minutes at 365F. Stir the meat every 10 minutes during cooking.

Nutrition: 184 calories, 18.5g protein, 1.3g carbohydrates, 10.8g fat, 0g fiber, 64mg cholesterol, 157mg sodium, 0mg potassium.

40. Pepper Pork Tenderloins

Preparation Time: 15 minutes

Cooking Time: 60 minutes

Servings: 2

Ingredients:

- 8 oz. pork tenderloin
- 1 tablespoon mustard
- 1 teaspoon ground black pepper
- 2 tablespoons olive oil

Directions:

1. Rub the meat with mustard and sprinkle with ground black pepper.
2. Then brush it with olive oil and wrap in the foil.
3. Bake the meat for 60 minutes at 375F.
4. Then discard the foil and slice the tenderloin into servings.

Nutrition: 311 calories, 31.2g protein, 2.6g carbohydrates, 19.6g fat, 1.1g fiber, 83mg cholesterol, 65mg sodium, 529mg potassium.

VEGETABLES

41. Brown Rice Casserole with Cottage Cheese

Preparation time: 15 minutes

Cooking time: 45 minutes

Servings: 3

Ingredients:

- Nonstick cooking spray
- 1 cup quick-cooking brown rice
- 1 teaspoon olive oil
- ½ cup diced sweet onion
- 1 (10-ounce) bag of fresh spinach
- 1½ cups low-fat cottage cheese
- 1 tablespoon grated Parmesan cheese
- ¼ cup sunflower seed kernels

Directions:

1. Preheat the oven to 375°F. Spray a small 1½-quart casserole dish with cooking spray. Cook the rice, as stated in the package directions. Set aside.

2. Warm-up oil in a large nonstick skillet over medium-low heat. Add the onion and sauté for 3 to 4 minutes. Add the spinach and cover the skillet, cooking for 1 to 2

minutes until the spinach wilts. Remove the skillet from the heat.

3. In a medium bowl, mix the rice, spinach mixture, and cottage cheese. Transfer the mixture to the prepared casserole dish. Top with the Parmesan cheese and sunflower seeds, bake for 25 minutes until lightly browned, and serve.

Nutrition: Calories: 334; Fat: 9g; Carbohydrates: 47g; Fiber: 5g; Protein: 19g; Sodium: 425mg; Potassium: 553mg

42. Quinoa-Stuffed Peppers

Preparation time: 15 minutes

Cooking time: 35 minutes

Servings: 2

Ingredients:

- 2 large green bell peppers, halved
- 1½ teaspoons olive oil, divided
- ½ cup quinoa
- ½ cup minced onion
- 1 garlic clove, pressed or minced
- 1 cup chopped portobello mushrooms
- 3 tablespoons grated Parmesan cheese, divided
- 4 ounces tomato sauce

Directions:

1. Preheat the oven to 400°F. Put the pepper halves on your prepared baking sheet. Brush the insides of peppers with ½ teaspoon olive oil and bake for 10 minutes.

2. Remove the baking sheet, then set aside. While the peppers bake, cook the quinoa in a large saucepan over medium heat according to the package directions and set aside.

3. Warm-up the rest of the oil in a medium-size skillet over medium heat. Add the onion and sauté until it's

translucent about 3 minutes. Put the garlic and cook within 1 minute.

4. Put the mushrooms in the skillet, adjust the heat to medium-low, cover, and cook within 5 to 6 minutes. Uncover, and if there's still liquid in the pan, reduce the heat and cook until the liquid evaporates.

5. Add the mushroom mixture, 1 tablespoon of Parmesan, and the tomato sauce to the quinoa and gently stir to combine. Carefully spoon the quinoa mixture into each pepper half and sprinkle with the remaining Parmesan. Return the peppers to the oven, bake for 10 to 15 more minutes until tender, and serve.

Nutrition: Calories: 292; Fat: 9g; Carbohydrates: 45g; Fiber: 8g; Protein: 12g; Sodium: 154mg; Potassium: 929mg

43. Greek Flatbread with Spinach, Tomatoes & Feta

Preparation time: 15 minutes

Cooking time: 9 minutes

Servings: 2

Ingredients:

- 2 cups fresh baby spinach, coarsely chopped
- 2 teaspoons olive oil
- 2 slices Naan, or another flatbread
- ¼ cup sliced black olives
- 2 plum tomatoes, thinly sliced
- 1 teaspoon salt-free Italian seasoning blend
- ¼ cup crumbled feta

Directions:

1. Preheat the oven to 400°F. Heat 3 tablespoons of water in a small skillet over medium heat. Add the spinach, cover, and steam until wilted, about 2 minutes. Drain off any excess water, then put aside.

2. Drizzle the oil evenly onto both flatbreads. Top each evenly with the spinach, olives, tomatoes, seasoning, and feta. Bake the flatbreads within 5 to 7 minutes, or until lightly browned. Cut each into four pieces and serve hot.

Nutrition: Calories: 411; Fat: 15g; Carbohydrates: 53g; Fiber: 7g; Protein: 15g; Sodium: 621mg; Potassium: 522mg

44. Mushroom Risotto with Peas

Preparation time: 15 minutes

Cooking time: 20 minutes

Servings: 2

Ingredients:

- 2 cups low-sodium vegetable or chicken broth
- 1 teaspoon olive oil
- 8 ounces baby portobello mushrooms, thinly sliced
- ½ cup frozen peas
- 1 teaspoon butter
- 1 cup Arborio rice
- 1 tablespoon grated Parmesan cheese

Directions:

1. Pour the broth into a microwave-proof glass measuring cup. Microwave on high for 1½ minutes or until hot. Warm-up oil over medium heat in a large saucepan. Add the mushrooms and stir for 1 minute. Cover and cook until soft, about 3 more minutes. Stir in the peas and reduce the heat to low.

2. Put the mushroom batter to the saucepan's sides and add the butter to the middle, heating until melted. Put the rice in the saucepan and stir for 1 to 2 minutes to lightly toast. Add the hot broth, ½ cup at a time, and stir gently.

3. As the broth is cooked into the rice, continue adding more broth, ½ cup at a time, stirring after each addition, until all broth is added. Once all of the liquid is absorbed (this should take 15 minutes), remove from the heat. Serve immediately, topped with Parmesan cheese.

Nutrition: Calories: 430; Fat: 6g; Carbohydrates: 83g; Fiber: 5g; Protein: 10g; Sodium: 78mg; Potassium: 558mg

45. Loaded Tofu Burrito with Black Beans

Preparation time: 15 minutes

Cooking time: 20 minutes

Servings: 2

Ingredients:

- 4 ounces extra-firm tofu, pressed and cut into 2-inch cubes
- 2 teaspoons mesquite salt-free seasoning, divided
- 2 teaspoons canola oil
- 1 cup thinly sliced bell peppers
- ½ cup diced onions
- 2/3 cup of black beans, drained
- 2 (10-inch) whole-wheat tortillas
- 1 tablespoon sriracha
- Nonfat Greek yogurt, for serving

Directions:

1. Put the tofu and 1 teaspoon of seasoning in a medium zip-top plastic freezer bag and toss until the tofu is well coated.

2. Heat-up the oil in a medium skillet over medium-high heat. Put the tofu in the skillet. Don't stir; allow the tofu to brown before turning. When lightly browned, about 6 minutes, transfer the tofu from the skillet to a small bowl and set aside.

3. Put the peppers plus onions in the skillet and sauté until tender, about 5 minutes. Lower the heat to medium-low, then put the beans and the remaining seasoning. Cook within 5 minutes.

4. For the burritos, lay each tortilla flat on a work surface. Place half of the tofu in the center of each tortilla, top with half of the pepper-bean mixture, and drizzle with the sriracha.

5. Fold the bottom portion of each tortilla up and over the tofu mixture. Then fold each side into the middle, tuck in, and tightly roll it up toward the open end. Serve with a dollop of yogurt.

Nutrition: Calories: 327; Fat: 12g; Carbohydrates: 41g; Fiber: 11g; Protein: 16g; Sodium: 282mg

SNACK AND DESSERTS

46. Cherry Stew

Preparation time: 10 minutes

Cooking time: 10 minutes

Servings: 6

Ingredients:

- ½ cup cocoa powder
- 1 pound cherries, pitted
- ¼ cup coconut sugar
- 2 cups water

Directions:

1. In a pan, combine the cherries with the water, sugar and the cocoa powder, stir, cook over medium heat for 10 minutes, divide into bowls and serve cold.
2. Enjoy!

Nutrition: Calories 207, Fat 1, Fiber 3, Carbs 8, Protein 6

47. Rice Pudding

Preparation time: 10 minutes

Cooking time: 45 minutes

Servings: 6

Ingredients:

- ½ cup basmati rice
- 4 cups almond milk
- ¼ cup raisins
- 3 tablespoons coconut sugar
- ½ teaspoon cardamom powder
- ¼ teaspoon cinnamon powder
- ¼ cup walnuts, chopped
- 1 tablespoon lemon zest, grated

Directions:

1. In a pan, mix sugar with milk, stir, bring to a boil over medium-high heat, add rice, raisins, cardamom, cinnamon, walnuts and lemon zest, stir, cover the pan, reduce heat to low, cook for 40 minutes, divide into bowls and serve cold.
2. Enjoy!

Nutrition: Calories 200, Fat 4, Fiber 5, Carbs 8, Protein 3

48. Apple Loaf

Preparation time: 10 minutes

Cooking time: 35 minutes

Servings: 6

Ingredients:

- 3 cups apples, cored and cubed
- 1 cup coconut sugar
- 1 tablespoon vanilla
- 2 eggs
- 1 tablespoon apple pie spice
- 2 cups almond flour
- 1 tablespoon baking powder
- 1 tablespoon coconut oil, melted

Directions

1. In a bowl, mix apples with coconut sugar, vanilla, eggs, apple pie spice, almond flour, baking powder and oil, whisk, pour into a loaf pan, introduce in the oven and bake at 350 degrees F for 35 minutes.
2. Serve cold.
3. Enjoy!

Nutrition: Calories 180, Fat 6, Fiber 5, Carbs 12, Protein 4

49. Cauliflower Cinnamon Pudding

Preparation time: 10 minutes

Cooking time: 20 minutes

Servings: 6

Ingredients:

- 1 tablespoon coconut oil, melted
- 7 ounces cauliflower rice
- 4 ounces water
- 16 ounces coconut milk
- 3 ounces coconut sugar
- 1 egg
- 1 teaspoon cinnamon powder
- 1 teaspoon vanilla extract

Directions:

1. In a pan, combine the oil with the rice, water, milk, sugar, egg, cinnamon and vanilla, whisk well, bring to a simmer, cook for 20 minutes over medium heat, divide into bowls and serve cold.
2. Enjoy!

Nutrition: Calories 202, Fat 2, Fiber 6, Carbs 8, Protein 7

50. Rhubarb Stew

Preparation time: 10 minutes

Cooking time: 5 minutes

Servings: 3

Ingredients:

- Juice of 1 lemon
- 1 teaspoon lemon zest, grated
- 1 and ½ cup coconut sugar
- 4 and ½ cups rhubarbs, roughly chopped
- 1 and ½ cups water

Directions:

1. In a pan, combine the rhubarb with the water, lemon juice, lemon zest and coconut sugar, toss, bring to a simmer over medium heat, cook for 5 minutes, and divide into bowls and serve cold.
2. Enjoy!

Nutrition: Calories 108, Fat 1, Fiber 4, Carbs 8, Protein 5

CPSIA information can be obtained
at www.ICGtesting.com
Printed in the USA
LVHW020704260421
685568LV00002B/62

9 781802 153040